Intermittent Fasting For Woman Over 50 Crash Course

A Modern Guide to Achieve a Rapid Weight Loss, Increase Energy And Detox Your Body, Promote Longevity And Support Your Hormones.

Anna Evans

© Copyright 2021 - All rights reserved.

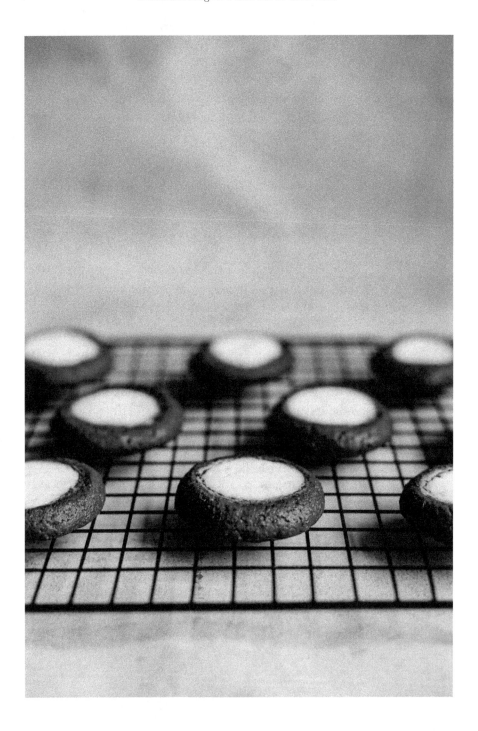

Table Of Contents

INTRODUCTION 8

CHAPTER 1. HISTORY OF INTERMITTENT FASTING 10

WHAT IS INTERMITTENT FASTING? 12

HOW DOES INTERMITTENT FASTING WORK? 12

CHAPTER 2. BENEFITS OF INTERMITTENT FASTING FOR WOMEN OVER AGE 50 14

REDUCTION IN THE RISK OF CANCER 14

REDUCES CARDIOVASCULAR DISEASE 16

SLOWS DOWN AGING PROCESS 17

INTERMITTENT FASTING FOR BETTER MENTAL AND MEMORY PERFORMANCE 18

INCREASE PHYSICAL ENERGY 18

INCREASE LONGEVITY 19

CHAPTER 3. INTERMITTENT FASTING FOR WOMEN OVER 50 22

WHY START INTERMITTENT FASTING AFTER 50? 22

ADVANTAGES OF INTERMITTENT FASTING FOR WOMEN OVER 50 25

TRICKS AGAINST HUNGER ATTACKS 29

CHAPTER 4. INTERMITTENT FASTING TYPES 30

24-HOUR FASTING 31

16/8 INTERMITTENT FASTING 31

THE WARRIOR DIET 32

ONE MEAL A DAY OMAD 33

36-HOUR FASTING 33

48-HOUR FASTING 34

EXPANDED FASTING (3-7 DAYS) 35

ALTERNATE DAY FASTING 36

FASTING MIMICKING DIET (FMD)...36

PROTEIN SPARING MODIFIED FASTING 37

CHAPTER 5. BREAKFASTS...38

1. BLUEBERRY-LEMON SMOOTHIE 38

2. QUINOA BERRY BOWL 39

3. BLUEBERRY MUFFINS..40

4. BAKED FENNEL 42

5. BROCCOLI RABE WITH LEMON AND CHEESE.................44

6. CAULIFLOWER FRIED RICE 46

7. AVOCADO DEVILED EGGS...48

8. FRESH FIG AND RASPBERRY COMPOTE...........................50

9. OVEN-ROASTED PEARS 51

10. HAWAIIAN-STYLE SNOW CONES 52

11. VANILLA YOGURT..53

12. BANANA FRITTERS...55

13. CHICKPEA SCRAMBLE BOWL 57

14. CHOCOLATE BREAKFAST QUINOA 59

15. BANANA QUINOA OATMEAL 61

16. AVOCADO SWEET POTATO TOAST 63

17. BANANA STRAWBERRY OATS 65

18. BLUEBERRY BANANA CHIA OATMEAL 67

19. SPINACH TOFU SCRAMBLE..69

CHAPTER 6. LUNCH... 72

20. CLASSIC STEAK 'N EGGS..72

21. HOMEMADE SAUSAGE, EGG, AND CHEESE SANDWICH.............................74

22. CHICKEN SAUSAGE CASSEROLE 77

23. CHEDDAR-CHIVE OMELET FOR ONE...79

24. STUFFED BELL PEPPERS...81

25. TUNA IN CUCUMBER...83

26. CHICKEN OMELET..85

27. LEMON BAKED SALMON 87

28. EASY BLACKENED SHRIMP...88

29. GRILLED SHRIMP EASY SEASONING 89

30. JAPANESE FISH BONE BROTH..91

31. GARLIC GHEE PAN-FRIED COD..92

32. STEAM YOUR OWN LOBSTER..94

33. THE BEST GARLIC CILANTRO SALMON..95

CHAPTER 7. DINNER... 98

34. SEAFOOD CASSEROLE 98

35. GROUND BEEF AND RICE SOUP..100

36. COUSCOUS BURGERS 102

37. BAKED FLOUNDER 104

38. PERSIAN CHICKEN..106

39. PORK SOUVLAKI...108

40. STUFFED BEEF LOIN IN STICKY SAUCE 109

CONCLUSION 112

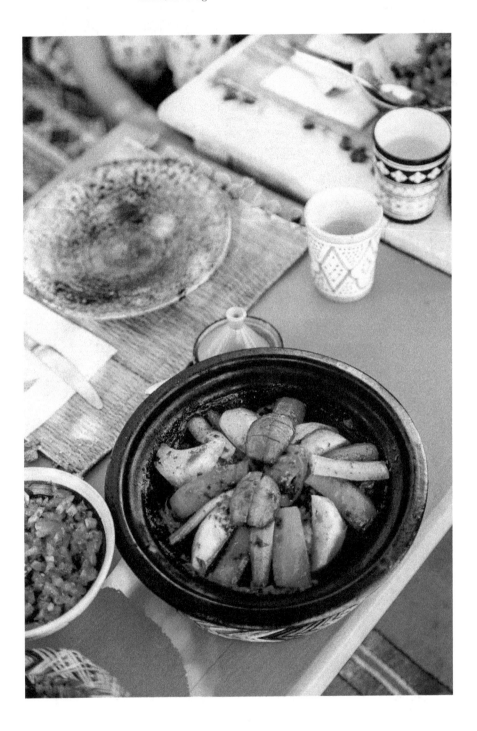

INTRODUCTION

You may have heard about Intermittent Fasting from your friends, or maybe some random talk show mentioned it as some fat loss miracle. You've overheard some women at the gym bringing it up during their chat about carb-cycling and protein shakes, but what is it? The name says it all. Intermittent-periods; fasting—being without food. What's so special about periods without food? Every time I say the word fasting to my relatives, they get this big fearful look on their faces as if I am starving myself and could die at any moment! Fortunately, you won't be starving yourself. It's not one of those fasts that last 30 days and have you drinking lemonade and spices.

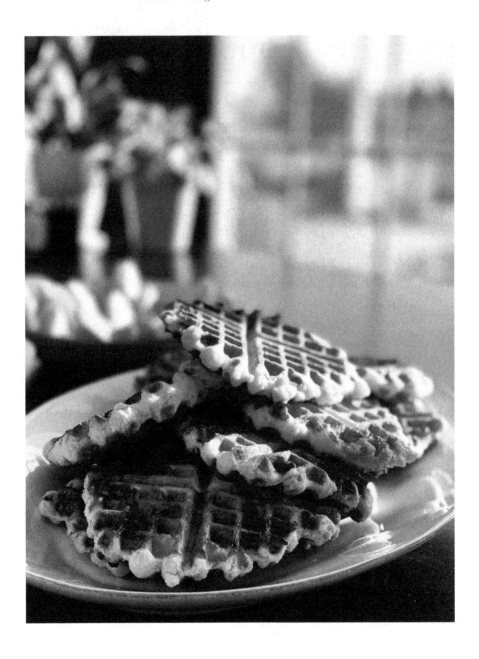

CHAPTER 1. HISTORY OF INTERMITTENT FASTING

When you feel the need to lose weight and cutting down your calories, you will find intermittent fasting the best way for sure. There are many ways by which you can reduce weight, but intermittent fasting or periodic fasting has many benefits apart from weight loss. Eating healthy, cutting down calories that are eating in a caloric deficit, and doing workouts will reduce weight. Here comes the question of how the idea of intermittent fasting came into being and who discovered it?

Fasting is an ancient ritual, which has been followed over the centuries by many cultures and religions. It is important to understand that fasting and starvation are two different things and shouldn't be mixed up. Starvation is a term used when the person has no idea about the availability of the meal, and there is a shortage of resources while fasting is avoiding the meals intentionally and the food is available.

Periodic fasting was used not just to cure the illnesses in ancient Egypt and Greece but also to prevent many diseases. Intermittent fasting was highly common in the middle Ages as people sought to enjoy its benefits. It was seen that intermittent fasting not only helps in reducing weight but also decreases insulin resistance. It is also used for the prevention of many diseases.

Intermittent fasting is the most common debate these days, so scientists are busy collecting intermittent fasting data. Studies conducted by Harvard have stated that fasting improves health, and those who practice intermittent fasting there are chances of increased life expectancy. This is quite obvious healthy individuals will survive longer because they will be physically active, and their body will be in the best state of health.

Intermittent fasting is both physical and religiously related. Many people practice intermittent fasting as part of their religion. Like Muslims, they fast in the holy month of Ramadan; Hindus observe different types of fasting according to their religion. Judaism has several common behaviors that include Yom Kippur, the truth of some. During the political times by a very famous leader Mahatma Gandhi at India's time of independence, Fasting was also observed.

In addition to controlling blood sugar, eating just one meal a day brings more benefits: reducing waist size and increasing muscle through the hormone HGH. Assuming the individual does not ingest non-protein foods, lowering blood pressure, improving lipid profile through lower LDL and higher HDL, reduced CRP or inflation, sound, even earlier, more significant over time as in any case, etc.

The concept of intermittent fasting has evolved with time. Starting from the point where it was considered starvation or due to insufficient sources, people used to stay hungry for a more extended period, the term fasting was identified. The definition of intermittent fasting has been changed from a period of fasting for hours or eating only one meal.

What Is Intermittent Fasting?

Intermittent fasting is described as an eating method that hovers between eating and fasting on a planned schedule. Several researchers have shown that this fasting method is very efficient for weight control and control of various kinds of diseases.

While several other diets focus on what you should eat, intermittent fasting focuses on what time to eat. Intermittent fasting restricts your eating plan to a specified period of the day, which, when followed, will make you lose weight, burn belly fat, and live a healthy life. There are several ways of doing intermittent fasting; yours is to study yourself and see the one that aligns with your health status and works best for you, then keep to it.

How Does Intermittent Fasting Work?

Even though there are several intermittent methods, the main routine of practicing all of them is to choose a pre-arranged period when you will eat and fast daily. An example is eating for 8 hours a day and fast for 16 hours, and you can also eat for five days of the weak and fast for the other two days (although both fasting days must not follow each other).

Intermittent fasting is different from the usual eating method because by eating three times a day together with snacks and not engaging in exercise, then you are only building your calories every time and not burning the fats storing in your body.

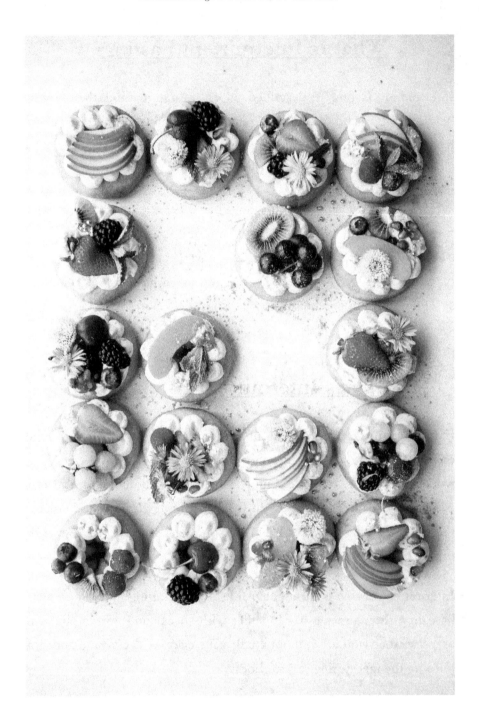

CHAPTER 2. BENEFITS OF INTERMITTENT FASTING FOR WOMEN OVER AGE 50

There are numerous benefits intermittent fasting has on the body of all humans and across all age groups. But in the course of this study, we are restricting our scope to women over 50. Some of these benefits are as follows:

Reduction in the Risk of Cancer

Intermittent fasting, which could also be referred to as mild caloric restriction, is very effective in the slowing down of fast-growing tumors that could lead to cancer.

Rous and Moreschi first discovered this benefit, and since then, it has gained wide recognition in the medical society. Restricting one's calorie intake also helps to boost the sensitivity of cancerous tumors to irradiation and chemotherapy.

Another benefit of intermittent fasting on women over 50 is the impairment of cancerous cells' metabolic process. This would make less energy available in the cell to function and most likely harm other cells.

Aside from that benefit, it serves to slow down, and if possible, shut down tumors, and it could help weaken them before treatments.

There is an action on transcription that boosts the effects of intermittent fasting against cancer. So, what is transcription? This is the process of copying information located in strands of DNA into molecular messengers called RNA.

The process is made possible by an enzyme known as RNA polymerase and many accessories of protein, which are classified as transcription factors. Some of these proteins include the forkhead box transcription factor (FOXO).

All the proteins play key roles in the process of metabolism, stress resistance, apoptosis (the programming process of cell death) as well as cellular proliferation (the process of cell growth).

Therefore, when this FOXO is activated during intermittent fasting, we could expect to see increased protection against carcinogenesis or tumorigenesis (the formation of cancer) and even the death of cancerous cells.

Another effect of FOXO's activation is increasing normal cells' resistance ability against stress, which could positively enhance the cells' longevity (and hence organisms).

Intermittent fasting may also play a key role in preventing cancer recurrence in women who had already been treated for cancer. Most times, these recurrences become more severe. Some cases of recurrence include stage IV breast cancer having a metastatic recurrence.

A study shows that women who carry out intermittent fasting exercise are less vulnerable to cancer recurrence (with a percentage of less than 36%). Intermittent fasting limits the amount of food that enters the body and reduces the amount of energy available to the cell.

Cells that are engaged in frequent restriction of Calories are known to less likely to develop changes that could lead to cancer. All these are owed to the positive and therapeutic effects of intermittent fasting on the cell and the immune system.

Reduces Cardiovascular Disease

Cardiovascular diseases (CVD) are known to have a very high mortality rate in women. Some of this CVD include; atherosclerotic cardiovascular disease (ASCVD), acute coronary syndrome (ACS), coronary artery disease (CAD), ischemic heart disease (IHD), etc.

Women above 50 have a higher chance of developing CVD, and although CVD affects both men and women, some risk factors increase the chances in women. These factors can be divided into two categories; modifiable and unmodifiable factors.

Among the unmodifiable factors are age, genetics, and gender. While the modifiable factors include hypertension, smoking, lack of physical exercise, obesity, poor diet, lipid metabolism disorder, diabetes, etc. Diabetes in women tends to increase the chances of a subtle heart attack without their knowledge.

Uncontrolled weight gain is the primary cause of obesity, which could lead to health disorders like diabetes, which increases the chances of developing CVD. Intermittent fasting has a great role it plays in insulin reduction, balancing heart rate, balancing high and low-density lipoprotein

Cholesterol (HDL and LDL). Also, it affects glucose levels as well as triglycerides, oxidative stress, and systemic inflammation.

Intermittent fasting boosts parasympathetic tone, which increases the variability of the heart rate. It does not only promote cardio-protection in overweight persons by enhancing weight loss; it works just as effectively in normal-weight individuals.

In other, for these positive changes to be lasting, one must continuously practice intermittently fasting, and the pattern or type of IF could depend on the preference of the individual.

<u>Slows Down Aging Process</u>

This is another benefit of intermittent fasting, and not until very recent years, the focus of intermittent fasting was to increase life span. This is because intermittent fasting was found to boost the body's general health and rejuvenate the body. The natural or even the induced aging process of the entire body is slowed down by doing this.

So, for women at 50 who, due to child-bearing and menopause, tend to age quicker than men, they can rely on strict adherence to intermittent fasting to slow down this process. The level of the effects of intermittent fasting varies from individual to individual.

However, its success is largely dependent on sex, age, genetic makeup, diet, environment, and other factors. Studies have shown that individuals who started intermittent fasting at a very young age have an increased lifespan (up to about 45%).

Individuals following a type of intermittent fasting experience strictly have a huge decrease in developing disorders that would be detrimental to their health. Hypertension, inflammation, obesity, dyslipidemia, and others, are lessened as a result of intermittent fasting. In fact, intermittent fasting is believed to have greater effects, which cannot be ascribed to only the reduction of calories.

Intermittent Fasting for Better Mental and Memory Performance

Intermittent fasting also enhances cognitive function and is very useful for boosting your brainpower. There are several factors of intermittent fasting, which can support this claim. First of all, it boosts the level of brain-derived neurotrophic factor (also known as BDNF), which is a protein in your brain that can interact with the parts of your brain responsible for controlling cognitive and memory functions as well as learning. BDNF can even protect and stimulate the growth of new brain cells.

Increase Physical Energy

This process influences not only your brain but also your digestive system. By setting a small feeding window and a larger fasting period, you will encourage the proper digestion of food. This leads to a proportional and healthy daily intake of food and calories. The more you get used to this process, the less you will experience hunger. If you are worried about slowing your metabolism, think again! Intermittent fasting enhances your metabolism; it makes metabolism more flexible, as the body now can run on glucose or fats for energy in a very effective way. In other words, intermittent fasting leads to better metabolism.

Oxygen use during exercise is a crucial part of the success of your training. You simply can't have performance without adjusting your breathing habits during workouts. VO2 max represents the maximum amount of oxygen your body can use per minute or kilogram of body weight. In popular terms, VO2 max is also referred to as "wind." The more oxygen you use, the better you will be able to perform. Top athletes can have twice the VO2 level of those without any training. A study focused on the VO2 levels of a fasted group (they just skipped breakfast) and a non-fasted group (they had breakfast an hour before). For both groups, the VO2 level was at 3.5 L/min at the beginning, and after the study, the level showed a significant increase of "wind" for the fasting group (9.7%), compared to just a 2.5% increase in the case of those with breakfast.

<u>Increase Longevity</u>

Autophagy is essential for the longevity of the organism. Autophagy has been shown to affect aging, which is why it plays such a large role in longevity. The reason for this is twofold. The first reason is that the cells that it acts in are often damaged or injured, and by way of autophagy, the disease or virus that is attempting to infect the organism is unable to spread, allowing the organism to continue living a relatively healthy life. This type of disease control increases the longevity of the organism.

The second reason is that autophagy is essential to maintaining the health of specific tissues and organs, which keeps them running smoothly and functioning at their best, which is also another factor that influences lifespan. If the organs and tissues are healthy, the organism as a whole will be healthy and will keep living.

In these two ways, autophagy plays a large role in the organisms' longevity and lifespan and their cells.

Autophagy can affect the quality of life of a person by maintaining their health and eliminating the disease. Inflammation in the short term helps to get rid of diseases, bacterial infections, and any sort of injury. By effectively eliminating disease and injury on time, the person's quality of life dramatically increases as their health is improved.

When it comes to the quality of life, autophagy has been shown to benefit mental health as well. Intermittent fasting, which induces autophagy, has been shown to decrease instances of depression and food-related disorders such as binge eating. Its benefits for weight loss also have been shown to improve body image, confidence, and overall self-satisfaction in adults who practice it for one month or more.

Other benefits of intermittent fasting include:

- Waistline reduction.

- Enhances psychological function.

- Prevention of neurodegenerative disorders, such as Parkinson's disease, stroke, etc.

- By reducing weight in obese women, intermittent fasting can dial down the symptoms of asthma.

- Tissue damages are reduced during intermittent fasting.

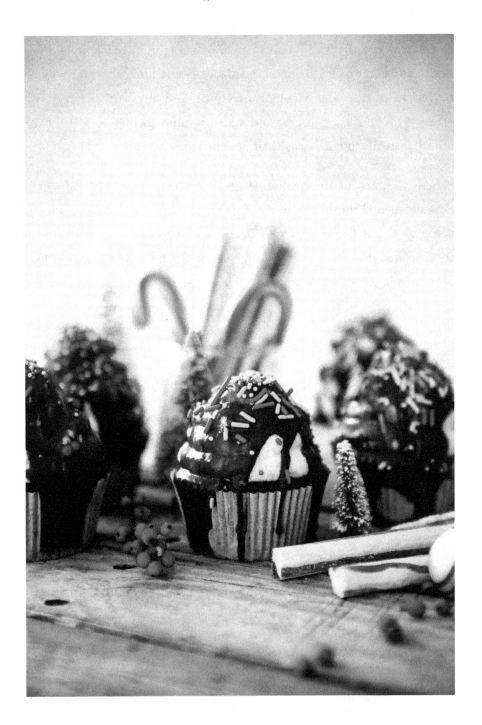

CHAPTER 3. INTERMITTENT FASTING FOR WOMEN OVER 50

According to researchers, intermittent fasting is beneficial for most people who eat during their daytime hours. Prolonged fasting differs from the usual eating style. If someone consumes 3 meals per day, including treats, and they don't work out, they operate on certain

Calories and don't burn their fat reserves at any time. Intermittent fasting allows our bodies to burn the reserved fat storage healthily; nine older women in ten have a form of chronic illness, and nearly eight in ten have more than one chronic disease. So, odds are, eventually, a person will get more. But to live a healthy life, there are measures one should take, and intermittent fasting is one of them.

Many of these chronic illnesses start from being overweight at an older age. The most important aspect of intermittent fasting is its weight loss assistance. Another research found that intermittent fasting induces less muscle loss than the more traditional form of daily restriction of calories. Bear in mind, though, that the primary explanation for its effectiveness is that intermittent fasting allows you to intake fewer calories overall. During your meal times, if you indulge and consume large quantities, you will not lose much weight at all.

Why Start Intermittent Fasting After 50?

Here, excess weight in women can cause these diseases, and intermittent fasting can help counteract them. Furthermore, intermittent fasting can help you control these aspects of living if you are over 50.

Hypertension

With age, blood vessels become less elastic when a person matures. This puts a strain on the mechanism that holds the body's blood. It may indicate why 2 in 3 women over the age of 50 have elevated blood pressure. The best approach to manage hypertension is to lose weight by intermittent fasting.

Diabetes

At least one in 10 women has diabetes. When you grow older, the odds of having the disease increase up. Heart failure, renal disease, blindness, and other complications may arise from diabetes due to excess weight.

Cardiac Condition

A significant source of heart attack is plaque formation in the arteries due to unhealthy eating. It begins in youth, and as one matures, it becomes worse. A large percentage of men and 5.6 percent of women have suffered from heart failure in the 40-58 age range in the U.S. Fasting and eating healthy is a good option to control any cardiovascular diseases.

Obesity

It might be dangerous for the health if one weighs too much for their height; it's not about getting a few extra pounds. More than 20 obesity chronic illnesses are correlated with stroke, asthma, arthritis, cancer, coronary failure, and high blood pressure. At least 30% of the older population is obese.

Arthritis

This condition of the joints was once directly attributed by physicians to the excessive wear and tear of time, and it sure is a cause. Yet biology and lifestyle are likely to have still much to do with it. A lack of physical exercise, diabetes, and becoming overweight may play a role in past joint accidents, too.

Osteoporosis

With old age, bones become weak, especially in women, which may lead to fractures. It impacts nearly 53.9 million Americans over 50 years of age. Some factors that will help: a balanced diet rich in vitamin D and calcium. Lose excess weight by fasting and daily weight-bearing activity, such as walking, jogging, and climbing stairs.

Tumor & Cancers

The greatest risk factor for old age is cancer. The disorder also impacts young adults, but between the ages of 46 and 54, your risk of getting it more than doubles. You can't influence a person's age or genes, but you have a choice in stuff like smoking or living an unhealthy lifestyle. With much of the study focusing on the beneficial impact that fasting has on cancer, fasting over varying periods has often helped older women decrease their risk of severe diseases. The study reported that fasting appears to suppress some cancer-causing pathways and can even delay tumor development.

Menopause

The classic indicators of menopause are hot flashes, insomnia, night sweats, mood swings, and vaginal dryness, burning, and itching. Heart failure and osteoporosis appear to escalate throughout the years of menopause. Often people start prolonged fasting to combat both the long-term and short-term symptoms of menopause. For several post-menopausal women, belly fat, not just for appearance but also for health, is a major concern. The decrease in belly fat resulting from intermittent fasting helped women minimize their likelihood of metabolic syndrome, a series of health conditions that enhance the risk of heart disease and diabetes for a post-menopausal female.

Advantages of Intermittent Fasting for Women Over 50

The benefits of intermittent fasting for women over 50 are limitless; some of them are mentioned here:

Decrease Insulin Resistance

Fasting is one of the most successful strategies to return the insulin receptors to a normal sensitivity level. Understanding the function of insulin plays is one of the biggest keys to learning about fasting and truly understanding every diet. About eating, insulin, the hormone that controls blood sugar, is formed in the pancreas and absorbed into the bloodstream. Insulin allows the body to retain energy as fat until released. Insulin creates fat because the fatter the body stores, the more insulin body makes or vice versa. The cycles during which a person is not eating allow the body time to reduce insulin levels, mainly during intermittent fasting, which changes the fat-storing mechanism. The mechanism goes in reverse, and the body loses weight as insulin levels decrease.

Autophagy is the amazing way cells "eat themselves" to get rid of dead cells and recycle younger parts. Autophagy is often the mechanism by which harmful pathogens, including viruses, bacteria, and other diseases, are killed. As the whole cell is recycled, another step in apoptosis. Your chance of cancer rises without this process when defective cells tend to multiply.

Intermittent Fasting Leads to Detoxification

Many of us have been subjected to contaminants from food and our climate in our lifetime. Many of these containments are processed in our bodies in fat cells. One of the most powerful methods to eliminate contaminants from the body is fasting and eating healthy.

The body's internal clock or Circadian Rhythm of the body controls virtually any mechanism in the body, and a chain of detrimental results will occur when it is disturbed. You adjust the circadian clock of the body while you take a rest from meals.

A Healthy Gut

It is one of the most important aspects of Fasting in that it provides a chance for the digestive tract and intestinal flora to reset. This is critical because the health of the body's digestive system regulates the immune system. There is even more proof that one's moods and emotional wellbeing are co-dependent on the gut microbiota. In recent studies of any area related to health and wellbeing, there has been a lot of hype on how one's gut flora might play an important part. The work of a more powerful immune system is important to a diverse microbiota, and it plays an important role in one's mental wellbeing. It also removes skin problems and reduces cancer danger.

Although the foods you consume have an immense effect on your intestinal health, periodic fasting in the digestive system can be another way to help grow the beneficial bacteria in the gut. Sugar and artificial goods disturb the equilibrium of your digestive tract between the beneficial and detrimental microbiota. Make sure to minimize packaged foods full of refined carbohydrates, sugars, and harmful fats that get the best outcome if you try intermittent fasting. Alternatively, switch to whole grains, plenty of organic vegetables and fruits, and good quality protein.

Intermittent fasting will work better by metabolic switching. Fasting contributes to lower glucose levels in the bloodstream. The body utilizes fat as an energy source instead of sugar after converting the fat into ketones.

Although it's not fasting, several physicians have recorded intermittent fasting advantages by permitting some easy-to-digest foods during the fasting window as fresh fruit. Modifications like this will also provide the essential rest for your metabolic and digestive system.

Losing Weight

It is expected that fasting helps accelerate the loss of excess weight. It also decreases insulin levels such that the body no longer receives the message to store more calories as fat during the state of fasting. Intermittent fasting may contribute to a self-activating decrease in calorie consumption by letting you consume fewer meals. Besides, to promote weight reduction, prolonged fasting affects hormone levels. It enhances noradrenaline or norepinephrine production, which is a fat-burning hormone, lowering insulin and rising growth hormone levels. Intermittent fasting can increase one's metabolic rate due to these changes in hormones. By encouraging one to eat less and activating ketones' production, intermittent fasting induces weight loss by adjusting all calorie calculation factors. In contrast to other weight loss trials, a study showed that this eating method would cause 3-8 percent weight loss in just weeks, which is a substantial percentage. People have lost 4 to 7 percent of their waist circumference; as per the same report, it is helpful for women dealing with menopause and unhealthy stomach fat that builds up over their organs and induces illness.

Other than insulin, during intermittent fasting are two important hormones, leptin and ghrelin. Ghrelin is the hormone of starvation that tells the body when it's hungry. Research shows intermittent fasting can reduce that ghrelin. There is also some evidence suggesting a rise in the leptin hormone, the hormone of satiety. That tells the body when it's full, and there's no more urge to eat.

People would be fuller quicker and hungry less frequently with less ghrelin and more leptin, which may lead to fewer calories eaten and, as a result, weight loss.

Tricks against Hunger Attacks

The best way to curb cravings is intermittent fasting. You don't eat for a certain number of hours each day, typically beginning at 6 am or later in this practice. You can have your main meal at noon and continue eating until 10 pm if you like, but it's generally recommended that you go without eating for 12-16 hours per day.

This practice of eating less often than normal and allowing your body to release stored sugar into your bloodstream is a proven method of curbing cravings and preventing hunger attacks. Intermittent fasting can also help curb the progress of aging, prevent heart disease, reduce cancer risk, and even boost immunity levels.

CHAPTER 4. INTERMITTENT FASTING TYPES

There are countless types of intermittent fasting. There are so many reasons why decide to follow an intermittent fasting lifestyle, and at least as many methods for doing it. Therefore, it is fundamental to set some basic definitions before we go deep in detail.

- Fasting – Giving up the intake of food or anything that has calories for a particular time frame. Normally, some non-caloric beverages and water are allowed.

- Intermittent Fasting – To fast intermittently by adding fasts into your regular meal plan.

- Extended Fasting – Fasting for a drawn-out time. It will, in general, be cultivated for a significant long time.

- Time-Restricted Feeding – Restricting your regular food usage inside a particular time window. This is meant to improve circadian rhythm and general wellness.

Generally, people who do intermittent fasting restrict their eating time and increase their fasting time. To have something like an actual fast, it would need to prop up for over 24 hours since that is the spot most of the benefits start to kick in.

First, let's have an overview of 10 of the main types of intermittent fasting, then we'll go deep into the 6 that better suit women after 50.

24-Hour Fasting

It is the fundamental technique of intermittent fasting—you fast for around 24 hours, and a short time later has a meal. Despite what the name may suggest, you won't actually go through an entire day without eating. Simply eat around the evening, fast all through the next day, and then eat again in the evening.

You can even have your food at the 23-hour check and eat it inside an hour. The idea is to make a very prominent caloric shortage for the day. Most of the benefits will be vain if you, regardless of fasting, binge and put on weight during the eating time frame.

Gradually and occasionally, you can decide to fast according to your physical condition and needs of the moment.

A fit person who works out constantly would require more eating time frames and a few fasting periods.

An overweight person who is sedentary and needs to lose some more weight could follow an intermittent fasting plan as long as they can until they lose the overabundance weight.

16/8 Intermittent Fasting

Martin Berkhan of Lean gains defined 16:8 intermittent fasting. It is used for improving fat loss while not having to go through an extremely demanding process.

You fast for 16 hours and eat your food inside 8. What number of meals you have inside that time length is irrelevant, yet whatever it is recommended to keep them around 2-3.

In my opinion, this should be the base fasting length to concentrate on reliably by everybody. There is no physical need to eat any sooner than that, and the restriction has many benefits.

Many people think it is more straightforward to postpone breakfast by two or three hours and then eat the last meal around early evening. You should not get insane, and it is demanding to observe the fast. The idea is simply to reduce the proportion of time we spend in an eating state and fast for a large portion of the day.

<u>The Warrior Diet</u>

Ori Hofmekler proposes the Warrior Diet. He talks about the benefits of fasting on blood pressure through hormesis.

The warrior diet not only improves your body's physical condition and resistance yet, moreover but also grows your mental attitude and outlook.

The Warrior Diet talks about old warriors like Spartans and Romans who used to remain on an empty stomach all through the day and eat in the evening. During daylight, they used to stroll around with 40 pounds of armor, build fortresses, and bear the hot sun of the Mediterranean, while having just a quick bite. They would have a huge supper around evening time consisting of stews, meat, bread, and many other things.

In the Warrior Diet, you fast for around 20 hours, have a short high power workout, and eat your food during a 4 hours window. Overall, it would merge either two minor meals with a break or one single huge supper.

One Meal a Day OMAD

One Meal a Day Diet, also called OMAD, simply consists of eating just one big meal every day

With OMAD, you regularly fast around 21-23 hours and eat your food inside a 1-2 hour time slot. This is remarkable for dieting since you can feel full and satisfied once the eating time comes.

It is unmatched for losing fat; be that as it may, not ideal for muscle improvement because of time for protein production and anabolism.

36-Hour Fasting

In the past, people would quite commonly go a couple of days without eating; they probably suffered and yet even thrived. Today, the average person can't bear to skip breakfast or go to bed hungry.

For over 24 hours is the spot where all the magic begins; the more you stay in a fasted state and experience hardship, the more your body is forced to trigger its supply systems that start to draw on fat stores, bolster rejuvenating microorganisms, and reuse old wrecked cell material through the system of autophagy.

It takes, at any rate, an entire day to see significant signs of autophagy. Yet, you can speed it up by eating low carb before starting the fast, rehearsing on an unfilled stomach, and drinking some homemade teas that facilitate the challenge.

For 36 hours, it's not really that annoying. You fundamentally eat the night before, don't eat anything during the day, go to sleep on an empty stomach, then wake up the next day, fast a few more hours, and begin eating again.

To make the fasting more straightforward, there are mineral water, plain coffee, green tea, and some homemade teas.

48-Hour Fasting

In case you made it to the 36-hour mark, why not give it a try to fast for a straight 48 hours.

It is only annoying getting through the change of habits. Once you overcome this obstacle, which generally occurs around your usual dinnertime, it gets a lot more straightforward.

The moment your body goes into an increasingly significant ketosis phase and autophagy starts, you will overcome hunger, feel very mentally clear, and have greater mindfulness and focus.

The most problematic bit of any complete fast is around the 24-hour mark. If you can make it to fall asleep and wake up the next day, you have set yourself prepared for fasting for a significant time with no issues from that moment onward. You essentially need to get over this hidden obstacle.

Going to bed hungry sounds disturbing; in any case, this is what a huge part of the world's population does daily. This could make you think about your own luck and feel thankful for having food anytime you want.

Expanded Fasting (3-7 Days)

48-hours fasting would give you a short ride in autophagy and some fat consumption. To genuinely get the deep health benefits of fasting, you would have to fast for three or more days.

It has been shown that 72-hours of fasting can reset the immune system in mice. However, studies on humans have not confirmed that conclusion; also, there may be some issues in prolonged fasting that are not under severe medical control.

Three to five days is the perfect time frame for autophagy, after which you may begin to see unwanted losses in bulk and muscle. Fasting for seven or more days is not generally suggested. Most people do not need to fast any longer than that since it may make them lose muscle tissue.

Fit people may want to focus on three-four of these expanded fasts every year, to propel cell recovery and clean out the body. Notwithstanding a healthy eating routine without any junk food, I do it anyway four times a year because of their tremendous benefits.

In case you are overweight or experience the negative effects of some illness, then longer fasts can really help you get back in health. Fast for three to five days, have a little refreshment break and repeat the plan until needed. I'll never say that enough; if you decide to go through this kind of longer fasting, be always sure of what you are doing and consult a doctor for any doubt.

Alternate Day Fasting

Alternate Day Fasting, as for the 5:2 Diet, is a very common type of fasting. Are they fully considered fasting, despite allowing the intake of 500/660 calories a day on fasting days? Well, yes, they are, since these limited amounts of calories are only intended to help extend perseverance.

To have a sporadic caloric intake will not enable the whole of the physiological benefits of fasting to fully manifest. It would limit a part of the effect. In any case, a strict limitation is important for both your physiology and mind.

Everybody can fast. It is just that someone cannot psychologically bear the weight of not eating. Fasting mimicking diets and alternate-day fasting in this respect.

Fasting Mimicking Diet (FMD)

The Fasting Mimicking Diet can be used every so often. Commonly, people who cannot actually fast, like old people or some recovering patients follow it.

Fasting mimicking diet has been shown to reduce blood pressure, lower insulin, and cover IGF-1, all of which have positive life length benefits. Regardless, these effects are likely an immediate consequence of the huge caloric restriction.

During the Fasting Mimicking Diet, you would eat low protein, moderate carb, and moderate fat foods like mushroom soup, olives, kale wafers, and some nut bars. The idea is to give you something to eat while keeping the calories as low as reasonable. In most cases, again, this is more about satisfying people's psychological needs of eating than the physical ones.

With zero calories would be just as effective, and it would keep up more muscle tissue by increasingly significant ketosis. To thwart the unwanted loss of lean mass, you can adapt the macronutrient taken in during Fasting Mimicking Diet and make them more ketogenic by cutting down the carbs and increasing the fats.

Protein Sparing Modified Fasting

Protein-Sparing Modified Fast (PSMF) is a low carb, low fat, high protein type of diet that helps to get increasingly fit quite fast while keeping muscle toned.

Lean mass is a significant matter of stress for healthy people, especially in case they are endeavoring to do intermittent fasting.

A catabolic stressor will, over the long term, lead to muscle loss; notwithstanding, the loss rate is a lot lower than people may imagine. To prevent that from happening, you have to stay in ketosis and lower the body's appetite for glucose.

PSMF is absolutely going to keep up more muscle than the fasting-mimicking diet. Yet, there's the danger of staying out of ketosis in case you are already eating many proteins preparing yourself for muscle catabolism.

CHAPTER 5. BREAKFASTS

1. Blueberry-lemon Smoothie

Preparation Time: 3 minutes

Cooking Time: 2 minutes

Servings: 2

Ingredients:

- ½ Banana

- 1 cup of Blueberries, frozen

- 1 cup of lemon yogurt

- ¼ cup of grape juice

- 1 teaspoon of Honey

Directions:

1. Using a blender, add in all the ingredients. Process until you obtain a smooth consistency.

2. Pour into two glasses and serve as a quick breakfast.

Nutrition:

- Calories 261 kcal Fat 2.5g Protein 6 g Carbs 57 g

2. **Quinoa Berry Bowl**

Preparation Time: 5 minutes

Cooking Time: 10 minutes

Servings: 4

Ingredients:

- 1 cup of Quinoa, cooked 1 tablespoon of Coconut oil

- 1 tablespoon of Coconut sugar ½ cup of Berries

- ½ cup (125 mL) Strawberries

- Coconut milk

Directions:

1. In a saucepan, cook the quinoa.

2. Drizzle coconut oil and add coconut sugar, mix well.

3. Add berries and strawberries.

4. Drizzle a little bit of coconut milk and serve.

Nutrition:

- Calories 224.7 kcal Fat 2.5 g Carbs 42.8 g

- Protein 4.4 g

3. <u>Blueberry Muffins</u>

Preparation Time: 5 minutes

Cooking Time: 25 minutes

Servings: 12

Ingredients:

- 2 Eggs

- 1 cup of Applesauce

- ½ cup of Maple syrup

- ½ cup of Avocado oil

- ½ cup of Vanilla extract

- 1 teaspoon of Cinnamon

- 1 teaspoon of Baking powder

- ¼ teaspoon of Baking soda

- 1 cup of whole Wheat flour

- 1 cup of Blueberries

Directions:

1. Preheat the oven to 325 °F.

2. In a bowl combine all the ingredients together, whisk well.

3. Add blueberries and scoop batter into 12 muffin cups.

4. Bake for 20-25 minutes.

5. When ready remove and serve.

Nutrition:

- Calories 217 kcal

- Protein 3 g

- Carbs 33 g

- Fat 8 g

4. <u>Baked Fennel</u>

Preparation Time: 10 minutes

Cooking Time: 50 minutes

Servings: 6

Ingredients:

- 3 Fennel bulbs

- 1 cup of Chicken broth

- ¼ cup of Gorgonzola cheese, crumbled

- ¼ cup of Panko bread crumbs

- Salt

- Pepper

Directions:

1. Cut the fennel bulbs in half lengthwise through the root end.

2. Put the fennel cut-side down in a skillet and add the chicken broth. Cover and simmer for 20 minutes.

3. Preheat oven to 375 °F. Place the cooked fennel bulbs in a baking dish, cut-sides up.

4. Mix the Gorgonzola with the breadcrumbs and divide the mixture evenly on the top of each fennel bulb.

5. Bake for 25 minutes, season with salt and pepper and serve hot.

Nutrition:

- Calories 75 kcal

- Fat 2 g

- Protein 3 g

- Carbs 12 g

5. <u>Broccoli Rabe with Lemon and Cheese</u>

Preparation Time: 5 minutes

Cooking Time: 15 minutes

Servings: 4

Ingredients:

- 1 quart of Water

- 1 teaspoon of Salt

- ½ cup of Broccoli rabe, trimmed

- 2 tablespoons of Olive oil

- 2 cloves of Garlic, chopped

- 1 tablespoon of Lemon juice

- Salt

- Pepper

- 2 tablespoons of Parmesan cheese

Directions:

1. Boil water; add salt and broccoli rabe. On low heat, simmer for about 8 minutes. Drain and shock under cold water and dry on paper towels.

2. Heat olive oil over medium-low heat and sauté the garlic for 5 minutes. Cut the broccoli rabe stems into 2 pieces and add to the garlic and olive oil. Sprinkle with lemon juice, salt, and pepper. Serve the Parmesan cheese at the table.

Nutrition:

- Calories 81 kcal

- Fat 8 g

- Protein 2 g

- Carbs 2 g

6. Cauliflower Fried Rice

Preparation Time: 10 minutes

Cooking Time: 10 minutes

Servings: 5

Ingredients:

- 1 Cauliflower head, halved

- 2 tablespoons of Sesame oil

- 2 Onions, chopped

- 1 Egg, beaten

- 5 tablespoons of coconut aminos

Directions:

1. Place a steam rack in the Instant Pot and add a cup of water.

2. Place the cauliflower florets on the steam rack.

3. Set the lid in place and the vent to point to "Sealing."

4. Press the "Steam" button and adjust the time to 7 minutes.

5. Release the pressure quickly.

6. In a food processor, add in cauliflower florets and pulse until grainy in texture.

7. Sauté the oil.

8. Stir in the onions until fragrant.

9. Stir in the egg and break it up into small pieces.

10. Add the cauliflower rice and season with coconut aminos.

11. Add in more pepper and salt if desired.

Nutrition:

- Calories 108 kcal

- Carbs 4.3 g

- Protein 3.4 g

- Fat 8.2 g

7. <u>Avocado Deviled Eggs</u>

Preparation Time: 10 minutes

Cooking Time: 6 minutes

Servings: 6

Ingredients:

- 6 Eggs

- 1 Avocado, pitted and meat scooped

- ¼ teaspoon of Garlic powder

- ¼ teaspoon of Paprika, smoked

- 3 tablespoons of Cilantro, chopped

Directions:

1. Place the eggs in the Instant Pot and add 1½ cups of water.

2. Close the lid and make sure that the vent points to "Sealing."

3. Select the "Manual" option and cook for 6 minutes.

4. Do quick pressure and release.

5. Allow the eggs to completely cool before cracking and peeling off the shells.

6. Beat the eggs and remove the yolk.

7. In a bowl, mix the yolk, paprika, avocado, and garlic powder. Sprinkle with pepper and salt.

8. Stuff the avocado-yolk mixture into the hollow egg whites.

9. Garnish with cilantro.

Nutrition:

- Calories 184 kcal

- Carbs 4.1 g

- Protein 9.6 g

- Fat 14.5 g

8. <u>Fresh Fig and Raspberry Compote</u>

Preparation Time: 3 minutes

Cooking Time: 17 minutes **Servings:** 4

Ingredients:

- ½ cup of Honey ¼ cup of Water 12 Mission figs, ripe

- 1 cup of Red raspberries 1 tablespoon of mint leaves, freshly chopped

Directions:

1. Mix honey and water together in a glass bowl and microwave on high for 20 seconds. Remove, stir, and let chill in the refrigerator.

2. Cut the figs into quarters and add them to the chilled honey syrup.

3. Add the raspberries and mint to the chilled syrup and let sit for 15 minutes in the refrigerator.

4. To serve, scoop the figs and raspberries onto four dessert plates.

Nutrition:

- Calories 242 kcal

- Fat 1 g Protein 2 g Carbs 62 g

9. <u>Oven-Roasted Pears</u>

Preparation Time: 6 minutes

Cooking Time: 55 minutes **Servings:** 4

Ingredients:

- 4 Bosc pears, ripe 1½ cups of Marsala wine

Directions:

1. Preheat oven to 450°F.

2. Place pears upright in a baking dish and pour the Marsala wine over them. Bake the pears for 20 minutes. Add water or more Marsala if the dish starts to get dry.

3. Baste the pears with the liquid in the dish and bake 20 minutes more.

4. Baste the pears again and bake longer until a knife inserted in a pear goes in easily.

5. Take out the pears and baste them several times as they cool. Serve at room temperature with a knife and fork.

Nutrition:

- Calories 217 kcal Fat 0.5 g Protein 1 g

- Carbs 31 g

10. <u>Hawaiian-style Snow Cones</u>

Preparation Time: 5 minutes

Cooking Time: 5 minutes **Servings:** 4

Ingredients:

- 4 tablespoons of Red bean paste 4 small scoops of Vanilla ice cream 4 cups of Shaved ice ½ cup of Syrup, flavored for snow cones

Directions:

1. Place a tablespoon of sweet red bean paste in the bottom of four insulated paper cones or cups.

2. Top the sweet red bean paste with a scoop of vanilla ice cream in each cone or cup.

3. Put a cup of shaved ice on top of the vanilla ice cream in each cone or cup.

4. Drizzle 2 tablespoons of flavored syrup over each shaved ice mound. Serve immediately.

Nutrition:

- Calories 259 kcal Fat 7 g Protein 3 g

- Carbs 48 g

11.   <u>Vanilla Yogurt</u>

Preparation Time: 10 hours

Cooking Time: 6 hours

Servings: 6

Ingredients:

- ½ gallon of Milk

- ½ cup of Yogurt starter

- ½ cup of Erythritol

- 1 tablespoon of Vanilla extract, pure

- 1 cup of Heavy cream

Directions:

1. Pour the milk into a crockpot and turn it on low for 3 hours.

2. Whisk in vanilla, heavy cream, and Erythritol and let the yogurt set.

3. While on low, cook for about 3 hours.

4. Whisk in your yogurt starter in 1 cup of milk. Add to the crockpot and mix well.

5. Set the lid in place and wrap the crockpot using two beach towels.

6. Let your wrapped crockpot sit for 10 hours while the yogurt cultures.

Nutrition:

- Calories 256 kcal

- Fat 21 g

- Carbs 6 g

- Protein 4 g

12. <u>Banana Fritters</u>

Preparation Time: 10 minutes

Cooking Time: 8 minutes

Servings: 2

Ingredients:

- ¼ cup of Almond flour

- 2 Bananas

- 1 teaspoon of Salt

- 1 teaspoon of Sesame oil

- 1 tablespoon of Water

- Powdered sugar

Directions:

1. Peel the bananas. Dice into bite-size pieces.

2. In a bowl, combine the flour, salt, sesame oil. Add 1 tablespoon of water. Stir until combined in a smooth batter.

3. Dip banana in the batter. Set on a tray. Place the tray in the freezer for 10 minutes.

4. Cover bottom of the fryer with parchment paper. Spray parchment with oil.

5. Preheat fryer to 350 °F.

6. Place bananas in the fryer. Spray bananas with a light coating of oil. Cook 4 minutes, flip over, spray oil on the other side. Cook 4 more minutes; until golden brown.

7. Transfer to a platter. Dust with powdered sugar.

Nutrition:

- Calories 242 kcal

- Fat 9 g

- Carbs 18 g

- Protein 5 g

13. Chickpea Scramble Bowl

Preparation Time: 10 minutes

Cooking Time: 10 minutes

Servings: Makes 2 bowls

Ingredients:

- ¼ of 1 Onion, diced

- 15 ounces of Chickpeas

- 2 Garlic cloves, minced

- ½ teaspoon of Turmeric

- ½ teaspoon of Black Pepper

- ½ teaspoon of Extra Virgin Olive Oil

- ½ teaspoon of Salt

Directions:

1. Begin by placing the chickpeas in a large bowl along with a bit of water.

2. Soak for few minutes and then mash the chickpeas lightly with a fork while leaving some of them in the whole form.

3. Next, spoon in the turmeric, pepper, and salt to the bowl. Mix well.

4. Then, heat oil in a medium-sized skillet over medium-high heat.

5. Once the oil becomes hot, stir in the onions.

6. Sauté the onions for 3 to 4 minutes or until softened.

7. Then, add the garlic and cook for a further 1 minute or until aromatic.

8. After that, stir in the mashed chickpeas. Cook for another 4 minutes or until thickened.

9. Serve along with microgreens. Place the greens at the bottom, followed by the scramble, and top it with cilantro or parsley.

Tip: if you don't prefer turmeric, you can omit it.

Nutrition:

- Calories 801 Kcal

- Proteins 41.5 g

- Carbohydrates 131.6 g

- Fat 14.7 g

14.   Chocolate Breakfast Quinoa

Preparation Time: 5 minutes

Cooking Time: 20 minutes

Servings: 1

Ingredients:

- ½ cup of Quinoa

- 1 ½ tablespoon of Cocoa

- 1 ½ cup of Soy Milk

- 1 ½ tablespoon of Maple Syrup

- 2 tablespoons of Peanut Butter

- Banana and strawberry slices (for topping)

Directions:

1. First, place the quinoa and soy milk into a medium-sized saucepan over medium-low heat.

2. After that, cook it for 13 to 15 minutes while keeping it covered.

3. Once the quinoa is cooked, stir in the peanut butter, sweetener, and cocoa powder to it.

4. Finally, transfer to a serving bowl.

Tip: instead of maple syrup, you can use brown rice syrup. You can even add cacao nibs to it. Also, you can add top to any berries.

Nutrition:

- Calories 650 Kcal

- Protein 19 g

- Carbohydrates 97 g

- Fat 22 g

15. <u>Banana Quinoa Oatmeal</u>

Preparation Time: 5 Minutes

Cooking Time: 10 Minutes

Servings: 1

Ingredients:

- ½ cup of Oats

- ½ cup of Quinoa, dry

- 2 Bananas, ripe

- ¾ cup of Almond Milk, light

- ½ teaspoon of Cinnamon, ground

- 2 tablespoons of Peanut Butter, organic

- 1 teaspoon of Vanilla

Directions:

1. To start, place the quinoa, oats, almond milk, cinnamon, and vanilla in a small saucepan.

2. Heat the saucepan over medium heat and bring the mixture to a boil.

3. Once it starts boiling, lower the heat and allow it to simmer for 10 to 15 minutes. Tip: the quinoa should have absorbed all the liquid at this time.

4. Next, fluff the quinoa mixture with a fork and then transfer to a serving bowl.

5. Now, spoon in the peanut butter and stir well.

6. Finally, top with the banana.

Tip: if you desire, you can add almonds to it for crunchiness.

Nutrition:

- Calories 386 Kcal

- Protein 11.7 g

- Carbohydrates 62.2 g

- Fat 11.8 g

16. <u>Avocado Sweet Potato Toast</u>

Preparation Time: 5 Minutes

Cooking Time: 10 Minutes

Servings: 1

Ingredients:

- 1 Sweet Potato, sliced into ¼-inch thick slices

- ½ of 1 Avocado, ripe

- ½ cup of Chickpeas

- 2 tablespoons of Sun-dried Tomatoes

- Salt & Pepper, as needed

- 1 teaspoon of Lemon Juice

- Pinch of Red Pepper

- 2 tablespoons of Vegan Cheese

Directions:

1. Start by slicing the sweet potato into five ¼-inch wide slices.

2. Next, toast the sweet potato in the toaster for 9 to 11 minutes.

3. Then, place the chickpeas in a medium-sized bowl and mash with the avocado.

4. Stir in the crushed red pepper, lemon juice, pepper, and salt.

5. Stir until everything comes together.

6. Finally, place the mixture onto the top of the sweet potato toast.

7. Top with cheese and sun-dried tomatoes.

Tip: if desired, you can add your choice of toppings.

Nutrition:

- Calories 452 Kcal

- Protein 19 g

- Carbohydrates 77 g

- Fat 11 g

17. <u>Banana Strawberry Oats</u>

Preparation Time: 10 Minutes

Cooking Time: 20 Minutes

Servings: 1

Ingredients:

- ½ cup of Oats

- 1 cup of Zucchini, shredded

- 1 tablespoon of Almonds, sliced

- ½ teaspoon of Cinnamon

- ½ of 1 Banana, mashed

- 1 cup of Water

- ½ cup of Strawberries, sliced

- Dash of Sea Salt

- 1 tablespoon Flax Meal

- ½ scoop of Protein Powder

Directions:

1. First, combine oats, salt, water, and zucchini in a large saucepan.

2. Cook the mixture over medium-high heat and cook for 8 to 10 minutes or until the liquid is absorbed.

3. Now, spoon in all the remaining ingredients to the mixture and give everything a good stir.

4. Finally, transfer the mixture to a serving bowl and top it with almonds and strawberries.

5. Serve and enjoy.

Tip: you can use any berries instead of strawberries.

Nutrition:

- Calories 386 Kcal

- Proteins 23.7 g

- Carbohydrates 57.5 g

- Fat 8.9 g

18. <u>Blueberry Banana Chia Oatmeal</u>

Preparation Time: 10 Minutes

Cooking Time: 10 Minutes

Servings: 1

Ingredients:

- ¾ cup of Rolled Oats

- 1 cup of Plant Milk

- 2 tablespoons of Chia Seeds

- ¼ cup of Blueberries

- ½ cup of Water 2 tablespoons of Agave Syrup

- ½ teaspoon of Cinnamon

- 1 banana, ripe and mashed

- Dash of Sea Salt 1 teaspoon of Vanilla

- 2 tablespoons of Peanut Butter

- 1 ½ tablespoon of Water

Directions:

1. To begin with, combine the chia seeds, sea salt, cinnamon, and oats in a mason jar until mixed well.

2. Next, pour in the hemp milk along with the banana, vanilla, and water to the jar. Stir again.

3. Now, mix the peanut butter with water in a small mixing bowl for 2 to 3 minutes.

4. Tip: The mixture should be creamy in texture.

5. After that, pour the creamy mixture over the oats and stir.

6. Then, place the Mason jar in the refrigerator overnight.

7. Add your favorite topping (¼-cup of blueberries) and enjoy.

Tip: if you desire you can add coconut flakes and or cacao nibs as a topping.

Nutrition:

- Calories 864 Kcal

- Protein 23 g

- Carbohydrates 107.4 g

- Fat 42.1 g

19. Spinach Tofu Scramble

Preparation Time: 5 Minutes

Cooking Time: 10 Minutes

Servings: 2

Ingredients:

- 2 Tomatoes, finely chopped

- ¾ cup of Mushrooms, finely sliced

- ½ red bell pepper, finely chopped

- 10 ounces of Spinach

- 2 tablespoons of Olive Oil

- 1 teaspoon of Lemon Juice, freshly squeezed

- ½ teaspoon of Soy Sauce

- 2 Garlic cloves, minced

- Salt & Pepper, as needed

- 1 pound of Tofu, extra-firm & crumbled 1 avocado (optional)

Directions:

1. First, take a medium-sized skillet and heat it over medium-high heat.

2. Once the skillet becomes hot, spoon in the oil.

3. Next, stir in the tomatoes, red bell pepper, mushrooms, and garlic.

4. Cook them for 2 to 3 minutes or until softened.

5. Now, lower the heat to medium-low and spoon in the spinach, lemon juice, tofu, and soy sauce.

6. Mix well and cook for a further 8 minutes while stirring occasionally.

7. Then, check the seasoning and add salt and pepper as needed.

8. Serve it hot.

Tip: instead of spinach, you can substitute kale, chard, or asparagus. If you want, you can add avocado slices.

Nutrition:

- Calories 527 Kcal

- Protein 36 g

- Carbohydrates 43 g

- Fat 29 g

CHAPTER 6. LUNCH

20. <u>Classic Steak 'n Eggs</u>

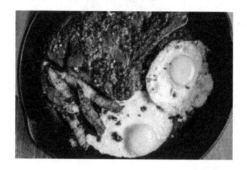

Preparation Time: 5 minutes

Cooking Time: 15 minutes

Servings: 4

Ingredients:

- 8 eggs

- 16-ounces of sirloin steak

- 4 tablespoons of butter

- 1 ripe avocado

- Salt and pepper to taste

Directions:

1. Melt 2 tablespoons of butter in a huge skillet.

2. Fry 4 eggs at a time until the edges are crispy.

3. While the second batch of eggs is cooking, cook the sirloin in another skillet (with the other 2 tablespoons of butter) until it's at least 160 °F.

4. Season eggs and steak well with salt and pepper.

5. Serve with slices of avocado.

Nutrition:

- Calories 480 kcal

- Protein 37 g

- Carbs 4 g

- Fat 37 g

- Fiber 3 g

21.   Homemade Sausage, Egg, and Cheese Sandwich

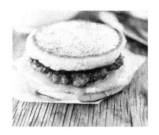

Preparation Time: 5 minutes

Cooking Time: 30 minutes

Servings: 1

Ingredients:

Muffin:

- 1 egg

- 1 tablespoon of coconut flour

- 1 tablespoon of almond milk

- ½ tablespoon of olive oil

- ½-teaspoon of baking powder

- Pinch of salt

Filling:

- 1 egg

- ¼-pound breakfast sausage

- 1 slice cheddar cheese

- ½ pounds ground beef

Directions:

1. Preheat oven to 400 °F.

2. Begin by mixing your muffin butter together first by cracking an egg in a bowl, then mixing in the rest of the ingredients.

3. Grease a ramekin and pour in the batter.

4. Bake for 15 minutes.

5. To get an egg that's the same size as your muffin, crack an egg in a ramekin and whisk.

6. Flavor with salt and pepper, then bake for 10 minutes.

7. For your sausage, just form the meat into a patty.

8. Heat a skillet, and then cook patty for 4-5 minutes per side.

9. When the muffins are ready, remove them from the oven and carefully slice them in half.

10. For a toasty muffin, stick in a toaster for a few minutes.

11. Build sandwich and top with a slice of cheese.

12. Eat!

Nutrition:

- Calories 460 kcal

- Protein 29 g

- Carbs 3 g

- Fat 37 g

- Fiber 0 g

22. <u>Chicken Sausage Casserole</u>

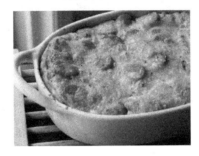

Preparation Time: 10 minutes

Cooking Time: 40 minutes

Servings: 4

Ingredients:

- 1 pound of chicken sausage

- 3 big eggs

- 2 cups of chopped tomatoes

- 2 cups of diced zucchini

- 1 ½ cups of cheddar cheese

- ½ cup of diced onion

- ½ cup of plain Greek yogurt

- 1 teaspoon of dried sage

- 1 teaspoon of dried mustard

Directions:

1. Preheat the oven to 375 °F.

2. Preheat a skillet until warm, and then add sausage.

3. When nearly all the pink is gone, put the zucchini and onion.

4. Cook until the veggies are softened.

5. Move skillet contents to a greased casserole dish.

6. In a separate bowl, mix eggs, yogurt, and seasonings together.

7. Lastly, mix one cup of cheese into eggs.

8. Pour into the casserole dish on top of the sausage and veggies.

9. Bake for at least 30 minutes until cheese has melted and starts browning.

10. Serve right away!

Nutrition:

- Calories 487 kcal

- Protein 19 g

- Carbs 4.8 g Fat 42 g Fiber 1.3 g

23. Cheddar-Chive Omelet for One

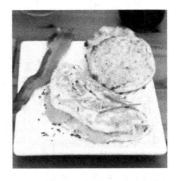

Preparation Time: 8 minutes

Cooking Time: 5 minutes

Servings: 1

Ingredients:

- 2 slices of cooked bacon

- 2 big eggs

- 2 stalks chives

- 2 tablespoons of sharp cheddar cheese

- 1 teaspoon of olive oil

- Salt and pepper to taste

Directions:

1. Heat oil in a skillet.

2. While that heats, chop chives.

3. Pour in eggs and sprinkle chives, salt, and pepper on top.

4. Wait until edges are beginning to set.

5. Crumble bacon on top and wait another 25 seconds.

6. Remove skillet from heat.

7. Sprinkle on cheese and carefully fold the omelet over.

8. Enjoy!

Nutrition:

- Calories 463 kcal

- Protein 24 g

- Carbs 1 g

- Fat 39 g

- Fiber 1 g

24. <u>Stuffed Bell Peppers</u>

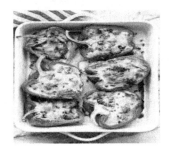

Preparation Time: 25 minutes

Cooking Time: 10 minutes

Servings: 4

Ingredients:

- 4 large yellow bell peppers

- 4 eggs

- 4 bacon strips

- 4 ounces of pork breakfast sausage

- 1 cup of shredded mozzarella cheese

- ½ cup of diced onion

- 1 tablespoon of minced garlic

- Couple of teaspoons of olive oil

- Salt and pepper to taste

Directions:

1. Preheat your oven to 275 °F.

2. Chop the tops off the peppers and hollow out the insides.

3. Set on a baking sheet and brush insides with a little olive oil.

4. Stick peppers in the oven.

5. Heat a skillet and cook bacon and sausage until nearly done.

6. Add onions and garlic.

7. Cook until onions have softened.

8. Take out the peppers and stuff.

9. Top with cheese and press down with a spoon, creating a little hollow.

10. Crack the eggs and put them inside of each bell pepper.

11. Turn oven up to 325 °F and put stuffed peppers in the oven for 10 minutes, or until eggs have reached the doneness you like.

12. Serve!

Nutrition:

- Calories 372 kcal Protein 27 g

- Carbs 1 g Fat 24 g Fiber 2 g

25. <u>Tuna in Cucumber</u>

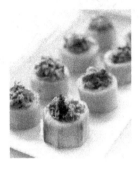

Preparation Time: 15 minutes

Cooking Time: 0 minutes

Servings: 6

Ingredients:

- 1 cucumber

- ½ celery leaf

- ½ red bell pepper

- 1 can of tuna

- Pepper and salt to taste

Directions:

1. Peel the cucumber and cut it into thicker circles. Make a hole in each piece.

2. Cut the celery and pepper into tiny cubes. Mix them with tuna.

3. Put 1 tablespoon of tuna mixture into cucumbers.

4. Add spices to taste and serve.

5. Enjoy!

Nutrition:

- Calories 109 kcal

- Total Fats 1.6 g

- Net Carbs 4 g

- Protein 1 g

- Fiber 5.4 g

26. <u>Chicken Omelet</u>

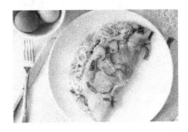

Preparation Time: 5 minutes

Cooking Time: 10 minutes

Servings: 2

Ingredients:

- 1 ounce of rotisserie chicken, shredded

- 1 teaspoon of mustard

- 1 tablespoon of mayonnaise

- 1 tomato, cored and chopped

- 2 bacon slices, cooked and crumbled

- 2 eggs 1 small avocado, pitted, peeled, and chopped

- Salt and ground black pepper, to taste

Directions:

1. Heat up a pan over medium heat, grease lightly with cooking oil.

2. Mix the eggs with some salt and pepper in a bowl and whisk.

3. Add the eggs to the pan and cook the omelet for 5 minutes.

4. Add the chicken, avocado, tomato, bacon, mayonnaise, and mustard to one-half of the omelet.

5. Fold the omelet, cover the pan, cook for 5 minutes and serve.

Nutrition:

- Calories 400 kcal

- Total Fats 32 g

- Net Carbs 4 g

- Protein 25 g

- Fiber 6 g

27. Lemon Baked Salmon

Preparation Time: 5 minutes

Cooking Time: 20 minutes **Servings:** 2

Ingredients:

- 12 ounces of filets of salmon 2 lemons, sliced thinly

- 2 tablespoons of Olive oil Salt and black pepper, to taste

- 3 sprigs thyme

Directions:

1. Preheat the oven to 350 °F.

2. Place half the sliced lemons on the bottom of a baking dish.

3. Place the fillets over the lemons and cover with the remaining lemon slices and thyme.

4. Drizzle olive oil over the dish and cook for 20 minutes.

5. Season with salt and pepper.

Nutrition:

- Calories 571 kcal Fat 44 g

- Fiber 2 g Carbs 2 g Protein 42 g

28. Easy Blackened Shrimp

Preparation Time: 10 minutes

Cooking Time: 6 minutes

Servings: 2

Ingredients:

- ½ pounds of shrimp, peeled and deveined

- 2 tablespoons of blackened seasoning

- 1 teaspoon of olive oil

- Juice of 1 lemon

Directions:

1. Toss all the ingredients (except oil) together until shrimp are well coated.

2. In a non-stick skillet, heat the oil to medium-high heat.

3. Add shrimp and cook 2-3 minutes per side.

4. Serve immediately.

Nutrition:

- Calories 152 kcal Fat 4 g Fiber 1 g Carbs 8 g

- Protein 24 g

29. Grilled Shrimp Easy Seasoning

Preparation Time: 5 minutes

Cooking Time: 5 minutes

Servings: 4

Ingredients:

Shrimp Seasoning:

- 1 teaspoon of garlic powder

- 1 teaspoon of kosher salt 1 teaspoon of Italian seasoning

- ¼ teaspoon of cayenne pepper

Grilling:

- 2 tablespoons of Olive oil

- 1 tablespoon of lemon juice

- 1 pound of jumbo shrimp, peeled, deveined

- Ghee for the grill

Directions:

1. Preheat the grill pan to high.

2. In a mixing bowl, stir together the seasoning ingredients.

3. Drizzle in the lemon juice and olive oil and stir.

4. Add the shrimp and toss to coat.

5. Brush the grill pan with ghee.

6. Grill the shrimp until pink, about 2-3 minutes per side.

7. Serve immediately.

Nutrition:

- Calories 101 kcal

- Fat 3 g

- Fiber 1 g

- Carbs 1 g

- Protein 28 g

30. Japanese Fish Bone Broth

Preparation Time: 5 minutes

Cooking Time: 4 hours **Servings:** 6-8

Ingredients:

- Fish head and carcass 4 slices ginger

- 1 tablespoon of lemon juice

- ½ leek, sliced Sea salt, to taste

- Water **Directions:**

1. Place the fish head and carcass into a large pot with cold water.

2. Bring to a boil and pour out the water.

3. Refill the pot with fresh water and add in the leek, sea salt, ginger, and lemon juice.

4. Simmer, covered, about 4 hours.

Nutrition:

- Calories 40 kcal

- Carbohydrates 0 g

- Fat 2 g

- Protein 5 g

31. <u>Garlic Ghee Pan-Fried Cod</u>

Preparation Time: 5 minutes

Cooking Time: 10 minutes

Servings: 4

Ingredients:

- 1¼ pound of cod fillets

- 3 tablespoon of Ghee

- 6 cloves of garlic, minced

- 1 tablespoon of garlic powder

- A pinch salt

Directions:

1. In a frying pan on medium-high heat, melt the ghee.

2. Add half the minced garlic.

3. Place the cod fillets in the pan and sprinkle with garlic powder and salt.

4. Cook until fish is a solid white color, about 4-5 minutes.

5. Then flip the fillets and add the remaining minced garlic. Cook until the whole fillets turn a solid white color, about 4-5 minutes.

6. Serve with the ghee and garlic from the pan.

Nutrition:

- Calories 160 kcal

- Carbohydrates 1 g

- Fat 7 g

- Protein 21 g

32. <u>Steam Your Own Lobster</u>

Preparation: 10 minutes **Cooking Time:** 10 minutes **Servings:** 4

Ingredients:

- 4 lobster tails 1 sprig parsley

Directions:

1. If the lobster tails are frozen, defrost them.

2. Before cooking, make a long slit in the underbelly of the lobster.

3. Fill a pot halfway with water. Place a steamer basket inside.

4. Once the water is boiling, place the lobster tails onto the steamer attachment.

5. Let boil for 8-9 minutes for fresh lobster and 10 minutes for defrosted lobster.

6. Garnish with parsley.

<u>Recipe Notes:</u>

If using fresh lobster, steam it for 8-9 minutes.

Nutrition:

- Calories 100 kcal Carbohydrates 0 g Fat 0 g

- Protein 24 g

33. <u>The Best Garlic Cilantro Salmon</u>

Preparation Time: 10 minutes

Cooking Time: 15 minutes

Servings: 4

Ingredients:

- 1 pound of salmon filet

- 1 tablespoon of butter

- 1 lemon

- ¼ cup of fresh cilantro leaves, chopped

- 4 cloves garlic, minced

- ½ teaspoon of kosher salt

- ½ teaspoon of freshly cracked black pepper

Directions:

1. Preheat the oven to 400 °F.

2. On a foil-lined baking sheet, place salmon skin side down.

3. Squeeze lemon over the salmon.

4. Season salmon with cilantro and garlic, pepper, and salt.

5. Slice butter thinly and place pieces evenly over the salmon.

6. Bake for about 7 minutes, depending on thickness.

7. Turn the oven to broil and cook for 5-7 minutes, until the top is crispy.

8. Remove salmon from the oven and serve immediately.

Nutrition:

- Calories 140 kcal

- Fat 4 g

- Fiber 2 g

- Carbs 3 g

- Protein 20 g

CHAPTER 7. DINNER

34. <u>Seafood Casserole</u>

Preparation Time: 20 minutes

Cooking Time: 45 minutes

Servings: 6

Ingredients:

- 2 cups of eggplant peeled and diced into 1-inch pieces

- Butter, for greasing the baking dish

- 1 tablespoon of olive oil

- ½ sweet onion, chopped

- 1 teaspoon of minced garlic

- 1 celery stalk, chopped

- ½ red bell pepper, boiled and chopped

- 3 tablespoons of freshly squeezed lemon juice

- 1 teaspoon of hot sauce

- ¼ teaspoon of Creole seasoning mix

- ½ cup of white rice, uncooked

- 1 large egg

- 4 ounces of cooked shrimp

- 6 ounces of Queen crab meat

Directions:

1. Preheat the oven to 350 °F. Boil the eggplant in a saucepan for 5 minutes. Drain and set aside.

2. Grease a 9-by-13-inch baking dish with butter and set aside—heat-up olive oil in a large skillet over medium heat.

3. Sauté the garlic, onion, celery, and bell pepper for 4 minutes or until tender. Add the sautéed vegetables to the eggplant, along with the lemon juice, hot sauce, seasoning, rice, and egg. Stir to combine. Fold in the shrimp and crab meat.

4. Spoon the casserole mixture into the casserole dish, patting down the top. Bake for 25 to 30 minutes or until casserole is heated through and rice is tender. Serve warm.

Nutrition:

- Calories 61 kcal

- Fat 2 g Carb 9 g

- Phosphorus 23 mg Potassium 178 mg Sodium 98 mg

- Protein 2 g

35. <u>Ground Beef and Rice Soup</u>

Preparation Time: 15 minutes

Cooking Time: 40 minutes

Servings: 6

Ingredients:

- ½ pound of extra-lean ground beef

- ½ small sweet onion, chopped

- 1 teaspoon of minced garlic

- 2 cups of water

- 1 cup of low-sodium beef broth

- ½ cup of long-grain white rice, uncooked

- 1 celery stalk, chopped

- ½ cup of Fresh green beans, cut into – 1-inch pieces

- 1 teaspoon of chopped fresh thyme

- Ground black pepper

Directions:

1. Sauté the ground beef in a saucepan for 6 minutes or until the beef is completely browned. Drain off the extra fat, then put the

onion and garlic in the saucepan. Sauté the vegetables for about 3 minutes, or until they are softened.

2. Add the celery, rice, beef broth, and water. Boil the soup, reduce the heat to low, and simmer for 30 minutes or until the rice is tender.

3. Add the green beans and thyme and simmer for 3 minutes. Remove the soup from the heat and season with pepper.

Nutrition:

- Calories 51 kcal

- Fat 2 g

- Carb 9 g

- Phosphorus 63 mg

- Potassium 198 mg

- Sodium 128 mg

- Protein 2 g

36. <u>Couscous Burgers</u>

Preparation Time: 20 minutes

Cooking Time: 10 minutes

Servings: 4

Ingredients:

- ½ cup of canned chickpeas, rinsed and drained

- 2 tablespoons of chopped fresh cilantro

- Chopped fresh parsley

- 1 tablespoon of lemon juice

- 2 teaspoons of lemon zest

- 1 teaspoon of minced garlic

- 2 ½ cups of cooked couscous

- 2 lightly beaten eggs

- 2 tablespoons of olive oil

Directions:

1. Put the cilantro, chickpeas, parsley, lemon juice, lemon zest, and garlic in a food processor and pulse until a paste form.

2. Transfer the chickpea batter to a bowl and add the eggs and couscous. Mix well. Chill the batter in the refrigerator within 1 hour.

3. Form the couscous mixture into 4 patties—heat olive oil in a skillet. Put the patties in the skillet, two at a time, gently pressing them down with a spatula.

4. Cook within 5 minutes or until golden and flip the patties over. Cook the other side within 5 minutes and transfer the cooked burgers to a plate covered with a paper towel. Repeat with the remaining 2 burgers.

Nutrition:

- Calories 61 kcal

- Fat 2 g

- Carb 9 g

- Phosphorus 133 mg

- Potassium 168 mg

- Sodium 108 mg

- Protein 2 g

37. Baked Flounder

Preparation Time: 20 minutes

Cooking Time: 5 minutes

Servings: 4

Ingredients:

- ¼ cup of mayonnaise

- juice of 1 lime

- zest of 1 lime

- ½ cup of chopped fresh cilantro

- 4 flounder fillets

- ground black pepper

Directions:

1. Preheat the oven to 400 °F. In a bowl, stir together the cilantro, lime juice, lime zest, and mayonnaise. Place 4 pieces of foil, about 8 by 8 inches square, on a clean work surface.

2. Place a flounder fillet in each square's center, then top the fillets evenly with the mayonnaise mixture. Season the flounder with pepper.

3. Fold your foil's sides over the fish, create a snug packet, and place the foil packets on a baking sheet. Bake the fish within 4 to 5 minutes. Unfold the packets and serve.

Nutrition:

- Calories 51 kcal

- Fat 2 g

- Carb 9 g

- Phosphorus 33 mg

- Potassium 98 mg

- Sodium 78 mg

- Protein 2 g

38. <u>Persian Chicken</u>

Preparation Time: 10 minutes

Cooking Time: 20 minutes

Servings: 5

Ingredients:

- ½ sweet onion, chopped

- ¼ cup of lemon juice

- 1 tablespoon of dried oregano

- 1 teaspoon of minced garlic

- 1 teaspoon of sweet paprika

- ½ teaspoon of ground cumin

- ½ cup of olive oil

- 5 boneless, skinless chicken thighs

Directions:

1. Put the cumin, paprika, garlic, oregano, lemon juice, and onion in a food processor and pulse to mix the ingredients.

2. Keep the motor running and put the olive oil until the batter is smooth. Put the chicken thighs in a large sealable freezer bag and pour the marinade into the bag.

3. Seal it, then put it in the fridge, turning the bag twice, within 2 hours. Remove the thighs, then discard the extra marinade.

4. Warm barbecue grill to medium. Grill the chicken within 20 minutes, turning once, until it reaches 165F. Serve.

Nutrition:

- Calories 321 kcal

- Fat 21 g

- Carb 3 g

- Phosphorus 131 mg

- Potassium 220 mg

- Sodium 86 mg

- Protein 22 g

39. Pork Souvlaki

Preparation: 20 minutes **Cooking Time:** 12 minutes **Servings:** 8

Ingredients:

- 3 tablespoons of olive oil 2 tablespoons of lemon juice

- 1 teaspoon of minced garlic 1 tablespoon of chopped fresh oregano ¼ teaspoon of ground black pepper

- 1 pound of pork leg, cut into 2-inch cubes

Directions:

1. In a bowl, stir together the lemon juice, olive oil, garlic, oregano, and pepper. Add the pork cubes and toss to coat.

2. Place the bowl in the refrigerator, covered, for 2 hours to marinate. Thread the pork chunks onto 8 wooden skewers that have been soaked in water.

3. Preheat the barbecue to medium-high heat. Grill the pork skewers for about 12 minutes, turning once, until just cooked through but still juicy.

Nutrition:

- Calories 61 kcal Fat 2 g Carb 9 g

- Phosphorus 33 mg Potassium 198 mg

- Sodium 98 mg Protein 2 g

40. <u>Stuffed Beef Loin in Sticky Sauce</u>

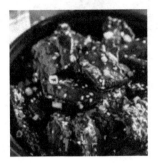

Preparation Time: 15 minutes

Cooking Time: 6 minutes

Servings: 4

Ingredients:

- 1 tablespoon of Erythritol

- 1 tablespoon of lemon juice

- 4 tablespoons of water

- 1 tablespoon of butter

- ½ teaspoon of tomato sauce

- ¼ teaspoon of dried rosemary

- 9 ounces of beef loin

- 3 ounces of celery root, grated

- 3 ounces of bacon, sliced

- 1 tablespoon of walnuts, chopped

- ¾ teaspoon of garlic, diced

- 2 teaspoons of butter

- 1 tablespoon of olive oil

- 1 teaspoon of salt

- ½ cup of water

Directions:

1. Cut the beef loin into the layer and spread it with the dried rosemary, butter, and salt.

2. Then place over the beef loin: grated celery root, sliced bacon, walnuts, and diced garlic.

3. Roll the beef loin and brush it with olive oil.

4. Secure the meat with the help of the toothpicks.

5. Place it in the tray and add a ½ cup of water.

6. Cook the meat in the preheated to 365 °F oven for 40 minutes.

7. Meanwhile, make the sticky sauce: mix up together Erythritol, lemon juice, 4 tablespoons of water, and butter.

8. Preheat the mixture until it starts to boil.

9. Then add tomato sauce and whisk it well.

10. Bring the sauce to a boil and remove it from the heat.

11. When the beef loin is cooked, remove it from the oven and brush it with the cooked sticky sauce very generously.

Nutrition:

- Calories 300 kcal

- Fat 23 g

- Fiber 2 g

- Carbs 8 g

- Protein 16 g

CONCLUSION

Intermittent fasting is not a new direction of dieting. In fact, people have been doing it since the beginning of time. Certain fasts, such as the Ramadan fast, Lent, etc., have been practiced since ancient times. Though based on beliefs and religions, these fasts are still forms of intermittent fasts and have similar positive effects as well. Intermittent fasting basically means eating at particular times during the day and fasting for the remaining time. So, for instance, if you have your breakfast at 8:00 a.m., you are supposed to fast until 8:00 p.m. The fasting period allows your body a resting period and leads to weight loss, glucose regulation, and various other benefits.

There exist a variety of intermittent fasts. Some of them are easy to do, while some are quite difficult for beginners. Regardless of the ease of an intermittent fast, it can still be one of the most difficult things you ever do if you have never fasted before. You need to regulate your diet cycle, which can be quite a task for many. Yet, it can't be compared to the grueling fact that you need to go 'hungry' for 8-10-12 or even more hours of the day. Eating one or two meals per day and going 'hungry' for the rest is especially difficult for people with busy schedules who are often accustomed to eating anything they find whenever they get the time. Such people avoid doing intermittent fasting because they believe that they cannot stick to the diet or will go hungry.